M000022359

Medicine Tracker

Keep Your Notes In One Place

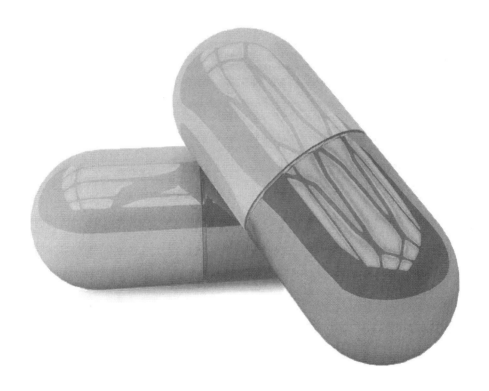

Life Log Books

Copyright © 2016 Uiri Press

First Printing

This book does not replace medical advice, nor is it intended for anything medical beside tracking.

All rights reserved. No part of this book may be reproduced or transmitted in any form or by any means, including but not limited to information storage and retrieval systems, electronic, mechanical, photocopy, recording, etc. without written permission from the copyright holder.

ISBN: 978-0692712115

Dedication

This book is dedicated to all the people on meds who need help keeping track of what they are taking, and to their caretakers who might need help too.

Important Information

My Name _____

My Phone Number _____

My Address _____

_____

Allergies _____

_____

Additional Important Information

_____

_____

My Doctor's Name and Phone Number

_____

_____

Medicine and Time Table

Date _Sample Page_

medicine	dose	time					
RX abc	5 mg	6am	10am	2pm	4pm	8pm	
RX xyz	20mg	7am	12pm	5pm			
RX grs	100 mg	6:30 am	12:30 pm	6:30 pm			
RX hij	500 mg	7:30 am	12:30 pm	5:30 pm			

Daily Check-In

How Do I Feel Today? _____
_____
_____
_____

I Had A Reaction To..._____
_____
_____
_____

I Need To Tell My Doctor About... _____
_____
_____
_____
_____

I Would Like To Change... _____
_____
_____
_____
_____

Medicine and Time Table

Date _____

medicine	dose	time					

Daily Check-In

How Do I Feel Today? _____

_____

_____

_____

I Had A Reaction To..._____

_____

_____

_____

I Need To Tell My Doctor About... _____

_____

_____

_____

_____

I Would Like To Change... _____

_____

_____

_____

_____

Medicine and Time Table

Date _____

medicine	dose	time					

Daily Check-In

How Do I Feel Today? _____

_____

_____

_____

I Had A Reaction To..._____

_____

_____

_____

I Need To Tell My Doctor About... _____

_____

_____

_____

_____

I Would Like To Change... _____

_____

_____

_____

_____

_____

Medicine and Time Table

Date _____

medicine	dose	time					

Daily Check-In

How Do I Feel Today? _____

_____

_____

_____

I Had A Reaction To..._____

_____

_____

_____

I Need To Tell My Doctor About... _____

_____

_____

_____

I Would Like To Change... _____

_____

_____

_____

_____

Medicine and Time Table

Date _____

medicine	dose	time					

Daily Check-In

How Do I Feel Today? _____

_____

_____

_____

I Had A Reaction To..._____

_____

_____

_____

I Need To Tell My Doctor About... _____

_____

_____

_____

_____

I Would Like To Change... _____

_____

_____

_____

_____

Medicine and Time Table

Date _____

medicine	dose	time					

Daily Check-In

How Do I Feel Today? _____

_____

_____

_____

I Had A Reaction To..._____

_____

_____

_____

I Need To Tell My Doctor About... _____

_____

_____

_____

_____

I Would Like To Change... _____

_____

_____

_____

_____

_____

Medicine and Time Table

Date _____

medicine	dose	time					

Daily Check-In

How Do I Feel Today? _____

_____

_____

_____

I Had A Reaction To..._____

_____

_____

_____

I Need To Tell My Doctor About... _____

_____

_____

_____

_____

I Would Like To Change... _____

_____

_____

_____

_____

_____

Medicine and Time Table

Date _____

medicine	dose	time					

Daily Check-In

How Do I Feel Today? _____

_____

_____

_____

I Had A Reaction To..._____

_____

_____

_____

I Need To Tell My Doctor About... _____

_____

_____

_____

I Would Like To Change... _____

_____

_____

_____

_____

Medicine and Time Table

Date _____

medicine	dose	time					

Daily Check-In

How Do I Feel Today? _____

_____

_____

_____

I Had A Reaction To..._____

_____

_____

_____

I Need To Tell My Doctor About... _____

_____

_____

_____

_____

I Would Like To Change... _____

_____

_____

_____

_____

_____

Medicine and Time Table

Date _____

medicine	dose	time					

Daily Check-In

How Do I Feel Today? _____

_____

_____

_____

I Had A Reaction To..._____

_____

_____

_____

I Need To Tell My Doctor About... _____

_____

_____

_____

I Would Like To Change... _____

_____

_____

_____

_____

Medicine and Time Table

Date _____

medicine	dose	time				

Daily Check-In

How Do I Feel Today? _____

_____

_____

_____

I Had A Reaction To... _____

_____

_____

_____

I Need To Tell My Doctor About... _____

_____

_____

_____

I Would Like To Change... _____

_____

_____

_____

_____

Medicine and Time Table

Date _____

medicine	dose	time						

Daily Check-In

How Do I Feel Today? _____

_____

_____

_____

I Had A Reaction To..._____

_____

_____

_____

I Need To Tell My Doctor About... _____

_____

_____

_____

_____

I Would Like To Change... _____

_____

_____

_____

_____

Medicine and Time Table

Date _____

medicine	dose	time					

Daily Check-In

How Do I Feel Today? _____
_____
_____
_____

I Had A Reaction To..._____
_____
_____
_____

I Need To Tell My Doctor About... _____
_____
_____
_____
_____

I Would Like To Change... _____
_____
_____
_____
_____

Medicine and Time Table

Date _____

medicine	dose	time					

Daily Check-In

How Do I Feel Today? _____

_____

_____

_____

I Had A Reaction To..._____

_____

_____

_____

I Need To Tell My Doctor About... _____

_____

_____

_____

_____

I Would Like To Change... _____

_____

_____

_____

_____

Medicine and Time Table

Date _____

medicine	dose	time					

Daily Check-In

How Do I Feel Today? _____
_____
_____
_____

I Had A Reaction To..._____
_____
_____
_____

I Need To Tell My Doctor About... _____
_____
_____
_____
_____

I Would Like To Change... _____
_____
_____
_____
_____
_____

Medicine and Time Table

Date _____

medicine	dose	time					

Daily Check-In

How Do I Feel Today? _____

_____

_____

_____

I Had A Reaction To..._____

_____

_____

_____

I Need To Tell My Doctor About... _____

_____

_____

_____

_____

I Would Like To Change... _____

_____

_____

_____

_____

_____

Medicine and Time Table

Date _____

medicine	dose	time					

Daily Check-In

How Do I Feel Today? _____

_____

_____

_____

I Had A Reaction To..._____

_____

_____

_____

I Need To Tell My Doctor About... _____

_____

_____

_____

_____

I Would Like To Change... _____

_____

_____

_____

_____

_____

Medicine and Time Table

Date _____

medicine	dose	time					

Daily Check-In

How Do I Feel Today? _____

_____

_____

_____

I Had A Reaction To..._____

_____

_____

_____

I Need To Tell My Doctor About... _____

_____

_____

_____

I Would Like To Change... _____

_____

_____

_____

_____

Medicine and Time Table

Date _____

medicine	dose	time					

Daily Check-In

How Do I Feel Today? _____

_____

_____

_____

I Had A Reaction To..._____

_____

_____

_____

I Need To Tell My Doctor About... _____

_____

_____

_____

_____

I Would Like To Change... _____

_____

_____

_____

_____

Medicine and Time Table

Date _____

medicine	dose	time					

Daily Check-In

How Do I Feel Today? _____

_____

_____

_____

I Had A Reaction To..._____

_____

_____

_____

I Need To Tell My Doctor About... _____

_____

_____

_____

_____

I Would Like To Change... _____

_____

_____

_____

_____

Medicine and Time Table

Date _____

medicine	dose	time					

Daily Check-In

How Do I Feel Today? _____
_____
_____
_____

I Had A Reaction To..._____
_____
_____
_____

I Need To Tell My Doctor About... _____
_____
_____
_____
_____

I Would Like To Change... _____
_____
_____
_____
_____

Medicine and Time Table

Date _____

medicine	dose	time					

Daily Check-In

How Do I Feel Today? _____
_____
_____
_____

I Had A Reaction To..._____
_____
_____
_____

I Need To Tell My Doctor About... _____
_____
_____
_____
_____

I Would Like To Change... _____
_____
_____
_____
_____

Medicine and Time Table

Date _____

medicine	dose	time					

Daily Check-In

How Do I Feel Today? _____

_____

_____

_____

I Had A Reaction To..._____

_____

_____

_____

I Need To Tell My Doctor About... _____

_____

_____

_____

_____

I Would Like To Change... _____

_____

_____

_____

_____

_____

Medicine and Time Table

Date _____

medicine	dose	time					

Daily Check-In

How Do I Feel Today? _____

_____

_____

_____

I Had A Reaction To..._____

_____

_____

_____

I Need To Tell My Doctor About... _____

_____

_____

_____

_____

I Would Like To Change... _____

_____

_____

_____

_____

_____

Medicine and Time Table

Date _____

medicine	dose	time					

Daily Check-In

How Do I Feel Today? _____

_____

_____

_____

I Had A Reaction To... _____

_____

_____

_____

I Need To Tell My Doctor About... _____

_____

_____

_____

I Would Like To Change... _____

_____

_____

_____

_____

Medicine and Time Table

Date _____

medicine	dose	time					

Daily Check-In

How Do I Feel Today? _____

_____

_____

_____

I Had A Reaction To..._____

_____

_____

_____

I Need To Tell My Doctor About... _____

_____

_____

_____

_____

I Would Like To Change... _____

_____

_____

_____

_____

_____

Medicine and Time Table

Date _____

medicine	dose	time					

Daily Check-In

How Do I Feel Today? _____

_____

_____

_____

I Had A Reaction To..._____

_____

_____

_____

I Need To Tell My Doctor About... _____

_____

_____

_____

_____

I Would Like To Change... _____

_____

_____

_____

_____

Medicine and Time Table

Date _____

medicine	dose	time					

Daily Check-In

How Do I Feel Today? _____

_____

_____

_____

I Had A Reaction To..._____

_____

_____

_____

I Need To Tell My Doctor About... _____

_____

_____

_____

_____

I Would Like To Change... _____

_____

_____

_____

_____

Medicine and Time Table

Date _____

medicine	dose	time					

Daily Check-In

How Do I Feel Today? _____

_____

_____

_____

I Had A Reaction To..._____

_____

_____

_____

I Need To Tell My Doctor About... _____

_____

_____

_____

_____

I Would Like To Change... _____

_____

_____

_____

_____

_____

Medicine and Time Table

Date _____

medicine	dose	time					

Daily Check-In

How Do I Feel Today? _____

_____

_____

_____

I Had A Reaction To..._____

_____

_____

_____

I Need To Tell My Doctor About... _____

_____

_____

_____

I Would Like To Change... _____

_____

_____

_____

_____

Medicine and Time Table

Date _____

medicine	dose	time					

Daily Check-In

How Do I Feel Today? _____

_____

_____

_____

I Had A Reaction To..._____

_____

_____

_____

I Need To Tell My Doctor About... _____

_____

_____

_____

_____

I Would Like To Change... _____

_____

_____

_____

_____

Medicine and Time Table

Date _____

medicine	dose	time					

Daily Check-In

How Do I Feel Today? _____

_____

_____

_____

I Had A Reaction To..._____

_____

_____

_____

I Need To Tell My Doctor About... _____

_____

_____

_____

_____

I Would Like To Change... _____

_____

_____

_____

_____

Medicine and Time Table

Date _____

medicine	dose	time					

Daily Check-In

How Do I Feel Today? _____

_____

_____

_____

I Had A Reaction To..._____

_____

_____

_____

I Need To Tell My Doctor About... _____

_____

_____

_____

_____

I Would Like To Change... _____

_____

_____

_____

_____

Medicine and Time Table

Date _____

medicine	dose	time					

Daily Check-In

How Do I Feel Today? _____

_____

_____

_____

I Had A Reaction To..._____

_____

_____

_____

I Need To Tell My Doctor About... _____

_____

_____

_____

_____

I Would Like To Change... _____

_____

_____

_____

_____

_____

Medicine and Time Table

Date _____

medicine	dose	time						

Daily Check-In

How Do I Feel Today? _____

_____

_____

_____

I Had A Reaction To..._____

_____

_____

_____

I Need To Tell My Doctor About... _____

_____

_____

_____

I Would Like To Change... _____

_____

_____

_____

_____

Medicine and Time Table

Date _____

medicine	dose	time					

Daily Check-In

How Do I Feel Today? _____

_____

_____

_____

I Had A Reaction To... _____

_____

_____

_____

I Need To Tell My Doctor About... _____

_____

_____

_____

I Would Like To Change... _____

_____

_____

_____

_____

Medicine and Time Table

Date _____

medicine	dose	time					

Daily Check-In

How Do I Feel Today? _____

_____

_____

_____

I Had A Reaction To..._____

_____

_____

_____

I Need To Tell My Doctor About... _____

_____

_____

_____

I Would Like To Change... _____

_____

_____

_____

_____

Medicine and Time Table

Date _____

medicine	dose	time					

Daily Check-In

How Do I Feel Today? _____

_____

_____

_____

I Had A Reaction To..._____

_____

_____

_____

I Need To Tell My Doctor About... _____

_____

_____

_____

_____

I Would Like To Change... _____

_____

_____

_____

_____

Medicine and Time Table

Date _____

medicine	dose	time					

Daily Check-In

How Do I Feel Today? _____

_____

_____

_____

I Had A Reaction To..._____

_____

_____

_____

I Need To Tell My Doctor About... _____

_____

_____

_____

I Would Like To Change... _____

_____

_____

_____

_____

Medicine and Time Table

Date _____

medicine	dose	time					

Daily Check-In

How Do I Feel Today? _____

_____

_____

_____

I Had A Reaction To..._____

_____

_____

_____

I Need To Tell My Doctor About... _____

_____

_____

_____

I Would Like To Change... _____

_____

_____

_____

_____

Medicine and Time Table

Date _____

medicine	dose	time					

Daily Check-In

How Do I Feel Today? _____

_____

_____

_____

I Had A Reaction To..._____

_____

_____

_____

I Need To Tell My Doctor About... _____

_____

_____

_____

_____

I Would Like To Change... _____

_____

_____

_____

_____

Medicine and Time Table

Date _____

medicine	dose	time					

Daily Check-In

How Do I Feel Today? _____

_____

_____

_____

I Had A Reaction To..._____

_____

_____

_____

I Need To Tell My Doctor About... _____

_____

_____

_____

_____

I Would Like To Change... _____

_____

_____

_____

_____

Medicine and Time Table

Date _____

medicine	dose	time					

Daily Check-In

How Do I Feel Today? _____

_____

_____

_____

I Had A Reaction To..._____

_____

_____

_____

I Need To Tell My Doctor About... _____

_____

_____

_____

I Would Like To Change... _____

_____

_____

_____

_____

Medicine and Time Table

Date _____

medicine	dose	time					

Daily Check-In

How Do I Feel Today? _____

_____

_____

_____

I Had A Reaction To..._____

_____

_____

_____

I Need To Tell My Doctor About... _____

_____

_____

_____

_____

I Would Like To Change... _____

_____

_____

_____

_____

_____

Medicine and Time Table

Date _____

medicine	dose	time					

Daily Check-In

How Do I Feel Today? _____

_____

_____

_____

I Had A Reaction To..._____

_____

_____

_____

I Need To Tell My Doctor About... _____

_____

_____

_____

_____

I Would Like To Change... _____

_____

_____

_____

_____

_____

Medicine and Time Table

Date _____

medicine	dose	time					

Daily Check-In

How Do I Feel Today? _____

_____

_____

_____

I Had A Reaction To..._____

_____

_____

_____

I Need To Tell My Doctor About... _____

_____

_____

_____

I Would Like To Change... _____

_____

_____

_____

_____

Medicine and Time Table

Date _____

medicine	dose	time					

Daily Check-In

How Do I Feel Today? _____

_____

_____

_____

I Had A Reaction To..._____

_____

_____

_____

I Need To Tell My Doctor About... _____

_____

_____

_____

_____

I Would Like To Change... _____

_____

_____

_____

_____

_____

Medicine and Time Table

Date _____

medicine	dose	time					

Daily Check-In

How Do I Feel Today? _____

_____

_____

_____

I Had A Reaction To..._____

_____

_____

_____

I Need To Tell My Doctor About... _____

_____

_____

_____

I Would Like To Change... _____

_____

_____

_____

_____

Medicine and Time Table

Date _____

medicine	dose	time					

Daily Check-In

How Do I Feel Today? _____

_____

_____

_____

I Had A Reaction To..._____

_____

_____

_____

I Need To Tell My Doctor About... _____

_____

_____

_____

_____

I Would Like To Change... _____

_____

_____

_____

_____

Medicine and Time Table

Date _____

medicine	dose	time					

Daily Check-In

How Do I Feel Today? _____

_____

_____

_____

I Had A Reaction To..._____

_____

_____

_____

I Need To Tell My Doctor About... _____

_____

_____

_____

_____

I Would Like To Change... _____

_____

_____

_____

_____

Medicine and Time Table

Date _____

medicine	dose	time					

Daily Check-In

How Do I Feel Today? _____

_____

_____

_____

I Had A Reaction To..._____

_____

_____

_____

I Need To Tell My Doctor About... _____

_____

_____

_____

I Would Like To Change... _____

_____

_____

_____

_____

_____

Medicine and Time Table

Date _____

medicine	dose	time					

Daily Check-In

How Do I Feel Today? _____

_____

_____

_____

I Had A Reaction To..._____

_____

_____

_____

I Need To Tell My Doctor About... _____

_____

_____

_____

I Would Like To Change... _____

_____

_____

_____

_____

Medicine and Time Table

Date _____

medicine	dose	time					

Daily Check-In

How Do I Feel Today? _____

_____

_____

_____

I Had A Reaction To..._____

_____

_____

_____

I Need To Tell My Doctor About... _____

_____

_____

_____

_____

I Would Like To Change... _____

_____

_____

_____

_____

_____

Medicine and Time Table

Date _____

medicine	dose	time					

Daily Check-In

How Do I Feel Today? _____

_____

_____

_____

I Had A Reaction To..._____

_____

_____

_____

I Need To Tell My Doctor About... _____

_____

_____

_____

_____

I Would Like To Change... _____

_____

_____

_____

_____

Medicine and Time Table

Date _____

medicine	dose	time					

Daily Check-In

How Do I Feel Today? _____

_____

_____

_____

I Had A Reaction To..._____

_____

_____

_____

I Need To Tell My Doctor About... _____

_____

_____

_____

I Would Like To Change... _____

_____

_____

_____

_____

Medicine and Time Table

Date _____

medicine	dose	time					

Daily Check-In

How Do I Feel Today? _____

_____

_____

_____

I Had A Reaction To..._____

_____

_____

_____

I Need To Tell My Doctor About... _____

_____

_____

_____

_____

I Would Like To Change... _____

_____

_____

_____

_____

Medicine and Time Table

Date _____

medicine	dose	time					

Daily Check-In

How Do I Feel Today? _____

_____

_____

_____

I Had A Reaction To..._____

_____

_____

_____

I Need To Tell My Doctor About... _____

_____

_____

_____

I Would Like To Change... _____

_____

_____

_____

_____

Medicine and Time Table

Date _____

medicine	dose	time					

Daily Check-In

How Do I Feel Today? _____

_____

_____

_____

I Had A Reaction To..._____

_____

_____

_____

I Need To Tell My Doctor About... _____

_____

_____

_____

I Would Like To Change... _____

_____

_____

_____

_____

Medicine and Time Table

Date _____

medicine	dose	time					

Daily Check-In

How Do I Feel Today? _____

_____

_____

_____

I Had A Reaction To..._____

_____

_____

_____

I Need To Tell My Doctor About... _____

_____

_____

_____

I Would Like To Change... _____

_____

_____

_____

_____

Medicine and Time Table

Date _____

medicine	dose	time					

Daily Check-In

How Do I Feel Today? _____

_____

_____

_____

I Had A Reaction To..._____

_____

_____

_____

I Need To Tell My Doctor About... _____

_____

_____

_____

I Would Like To Change... _____

_____

_____

_____

_____

_____

Medicine and Time Table

Date _____

medicine	dose	time					

Daily Check-In

How Do I Feel Today? _____
_____
_____
_____

I Had A Reaction To..._____
_____
_____
_____

I Need To Tell My Doctor About... _____
_____
_____
_____

I Would Like To Change... _____
_____
_____
_____
_____

Medicine and Time Table

Date _____

medicine	dose	time					

Daily Check-In

How Do I Feel Today? _____

_____

_____

_____

I Had A Reaction To..._____

_____

_____

_____

I Need To Tell My Doctor About... _____

_____

_____

_____

_____

I Would Like To Change... _____

_____

_____

_____

_____

_____

Medicine and Time Table

Date _____

medicine	dose	time					

Daily Check-In

How Do I Feel Today? _____

_____

_____

_____

I Had A Reaction To..._____

_____

_____

_____

I Need To Tell My Doctor About... _____

_____

_____

_____

_____

I Would Like To Change... _____

_____

_____

_____

_____

_____

Medicine and Time Table

Date _____

medicine	dose	time					

Daily Check-In

How Do I Feel Today? _____

_____

_____

_____

I Had A Reaction To..._____

_____

_____

_____

I Need To Tell My Doctor About... _____

_____

_____

_____

_____

I Would Like To Change... _____

_____

_____

_____

_____

_____

Medicine and Time Table

Date _____

medicine	dose	time					

Daily Check-In

How Do I Feel Today? _____

_____

_____

_____

I Had A Reaction To... _____

_____

_____

_____

I Need To Tell My Doctor About... _____

_____

_____

_____

_____

I Would Like To Change... _____

_____

_____

_____

_____

Medicine and Time Table

Date _____

medicine	dose	time					

Daily Check-In

How Do I Feel Today? _____

_____

_____

_____

I Had A Reaction To..._____

_____

_____

_____

I Need To Tell My Doctor About... _____

_____

_____

_____

I Would Like To Change... _____

_____

_____

_____

_____

Medicine and Time Table

Date _____

medicine	dose	time					

Made in the USA
Columbia, SC
22 November 2020

25231992R00076